Recognising Clinical Depression

A Quick Snapshot of

Symptoms, Causes and Treatments

N. I. Nwokolo

N. I. Nwokolo

ISBN-13:978-1721592463

ISBN-10:1721592466

For my beloved father, with deepest thanks.

PREFACE

We all have our 'down' days occasionally, but clinical depression is quite a different ballgame; its persistent and sometimes severe symptoms can bring about a significant deterioration in quality of life, impairments in day-to-day functioning, and even risk to life. It is a surprisingly common disorder. Up to 20% of people will suffer from depression at some point in their lifetime.

Suffering from depression, or watching a loved one suffer from it, can be a very distressing and even frightening experience. There remains a certain amount of perceived stigma around psychiatric illness, although this is improving significantly in the UK, with many celebrities and public figures speaking out in recent years about their own mental health struggles.

Identifying a mental health disorder, or what one thinks it could be, is the crucial first step in seeking a solution. Symptoms and signs of clinical depression, as described by the WHO's International Classification of Disorders, have been listed here. Known causes of depression and contributing factors have also been touched on briefly; it is natural for a depressed person or those close to them to wonder why this has happened to them in particular.

A very brief summary of treatments for depression, as recommended by the National Institute for Health and Care Excellence (NICE), is also provided. The book's references and a few mental health websites are provided at the end for further reading.

Like other psychiatric disorders, depression is believed to result from the interplay of multiple contributing factors, rather than just a single cause. These factors can be biological, psychological, or social in nature. A person might inherit a genetic tendency to suffer from depression (biological), and have low emotional resilience as a result of poor bonding with a parent in their childhood (psychological), and this could lead to biological alterations in their brain functioning and later difficulties in regulating their stress levels. As a result of these underlying factors, they might be more likely than other people to suffer a depressive episode triggered by difficult circumstances such as bullying at school, problems at work, or a difficult marriage (social).

Factors contributing to mental health problems can also be categorized as predisposing, precipitating or perpetuating. Inheriting a genetic tendency to develop depression is a *predisposing* factor, stressful life events often *precipitate* a depressive episode, and ongoing stresses can *perpetuate* the symptoms.

The seeking of psychiatric treatment is sometimes avoided or delayed due to stigma, fear, or even a failure to recognize that there is a mental health disorder. In some cases, by the time treatment can no longer be avoided, symptoms may have become quite severe.

The treatments required, or if treatment is sought at

all, will depend on the severity of symptoms and the extent to which an individual's functioning is impaired. In the UK the usual first port of call for someone seeking treatment for depression is the general practitioner (GP). Many cases of depression can be managed by the GP and/or community psychological services without requiring referral to a psychiatrist; mild depression may only require psychological treatments such as cognitive behavioural therapy (CBT) and monitoring by the GP.

Even where psychiatric referral is needed, only a tiny proportion of people with depression will ever require admission to a psychiatric ward. The vast majority are treated as outpatients. With the increased emphasis on psychiatric home treatment teams in recent years, even some individuals whose illness severity would have seen them admitted to hospital in the not-too-distant past are now being treated at home. In addition to psychological treatments, there is a wide range of antidepressants and other treatments available nowadays, with demonstrated effectiveness and fewer side-effects than earlier ones.

It is hoped that in demystifying depression to some extent for people who have not had training in mental health, including young people, a certain amount of anxiety will be dispelled, and many will feel encouraged and empowered to seek appropriate treatment where required.

N. I. Nwokolo

CONTENTS

Page

SIGNS AND SYMPTOMS

The central symptom of depression is a low (depressed) mood. Two other key features that often feature strongly are a sense of fatigue (loss of energy) and loss of pleasure in activities..

The International Classification of Diseases (ICD-10) provides the following characteristic symptoms of depression:

A persistent low mood of at least 2 weeks (although in occasional cases of acute onset it can be less)

Loss of interest and enjoyment

Mood may be unresponsive to experiences

Reduced energy

Reduced activity

Poor concentration

Reduced self-esteem and confidence

Feelings of guilt and unworthiness

Feelings of hopelessness

Feelings of worthlessness

Pessimistic views of the future

Ideas or acts of self-harm or suicide

Disturbed sleep (especially early morning wakening, but also initial insomnia, frequent waking and non-restful sleep)

Reduced appetite, sometimes with significant weight loss

Mood may be lower in the morning and improve as the day progresses (diurnal variation)

Slowing of movement and thinking processes (psychomotor retardation, which can progress to a stupor in very severe cases)

In some cases:
Anxiety and agitation
Irritability
Increase of existing phobias, obsessions and hypochondria
Increased intake of alcohol

In a number of cases, usually when severe:
Delusional ideas, which usually centre around sin, poverty or imminent disaster, for which the sufferer might feel they are personally responsible.

Auditory hallucinations (basically hearing noises or voices others cannot) which are usually in the form of defamatory or accusatory voices.

Olfactory hallucinations (smelling things others cannot), often of rotting filth or decomposing flesh.

Not everyone suffers from depression in exactly the same way, or experiences all the symptoms listed. Some people may even have the illness without actively feeling sad.

Depression can be mild, moderate or severe, depending on the number and severity of symptoms and levels of impairment of day-to-day functioning.

With mild depression, there may be a certain degree of difficulty in coping with day-to-day activities such as work, school, housework and socializing, but the individual does continue to function in these areas.

In moderate depression, there is considerable difficulty in continuing to carry out daily activities.

In severe depression, the sufferer is generally rendered unable to cope with their activities. They are usually extremely distressed or agitated, or they may become exceptionally slowed down in their thinking, movement and general functioning (psychomotor retardation). Self-neglect and neglect of daily chores may occur.

Some people experience what is described as 'atypical depression,' which features excessive sleep, excessive eating, significant fatigue and marked anxiety. The depression here tends to be moderately severe. The mood can vary, and may be responsive to positive experiences.

For a diagnosis of depression, the ICD-10 requires at least four symptoms to be present, with at least two of the three key ones (low mood, loss of interest/pleasure and loss of energy).

The National Institute of Health and Care Excellence (NICE) has recommended two questions that can be used as initial screening at the first assessment of someone suspected to be depressed (summarized below):

- Have you felt **down, depressed** or **hopeless** in the last month?

- In the last month, have you found **little interest or pleasure** in doing things?

Further assessment is recommended if there is a positive response to either or both questions.

Depression as a disorder can be very insidious; it is quite possible to rumble on functioning at a sub-par level for years without realizing there is a mental health issue present.

CAUSATIVE AND CONTRIBUTING FACTORS

BIOLOGICAL

o A genetic predisposition to depression (inherited tendency), believed to be linked to multiple genes

o An adverse environment in the womb before birth, leading to biological alterations in brain functioning and later difficulties in stress regulation

o Longstanding disruption to the body's stress regulation mechanisms controlled by hormonal interaction between the hypothalamus, pituitary and adrenal glands (HPA axis), as a result of adverse early experiences

o Reduced function of brain neurotransmitters (chemicals such as serotonin, noradrenaline and dopamine that transmit signals between nerve cells in the brain)

o Heightened inflammation in the body (can be triggered by stress, infections, poor diet and other causes)

o Organic causes (physical health problems) such as diabetes mellitus, rheumatoid arthritis, thyroid disease, Cushing's disease, Parkinson's disease, and cancer

o Changes in immune function

o Some medications

o Alcohol and other substance misuse

o Female gender

o Recent childbirth.

PSYCHOLOGICAL

o Individual personality or temperament (for example pre-existing high levels of anxiety, high neuroticism, a strong need for approval, and other personality difficulties)

o Negative thinking styles

o Other mental health disorders, such as bipolar affective disorder, anxiety disorders, schizophrenia and emotionally unstable personality disorder

SOCIAL

o Adverse or traumatic experiences in childhood such as bullying, parental break-ups, loss of, or separation from parents (these can cause disruptions to internal stress regulation mechanisms, resulting in low emotional resilience and increased sensitivity to later stress)

o Impaired maternal attachment

o Deprivation of maternal affection though loss or separation

o Disruption of parental, familial, marital and other social relationships

o Family discord

o Dysfunctional parenting styles

o Physical, emotional and sexual abuse

o Traumatic life events such as bereavement, relationship break-up or loss of employment

o Chronic stressful situations such as unemployment, financial difficulties, problems at work, marital difficulties, or experiencing prejudice

o Low socioeconomic status (low levels of education, employment and income) o Social isolation and lack of social support, particularly a confiding relationship.

TREATMENTS

A thorough psychiatric assessment will need to be carried out in each case, including a detailed history covering psychiatric symptoms, difficulties with functioning, past and present psychiatric and medical problems, family history, early development, social history, alcohol and substance use, and other issues.

Because medical illnesses can be a cause of depression, a physical assessment including routine blood tests and other investigations is generally requested. The treatment of any medical disorders will need to be arranged, through the GP or referral to relevant specialists.

Once depression has been diagnosed, the UK's National Institute for Health and Care Excellence (NICE) recommends the treatments below.

Mild depression:

'Low-intensity' psychological or psychosocial interventions such as:

- o Information on sleep hygiene (measures to improve sleep pattern), if required

- o Guided self-help, computerised or group programmes based on Cognitive Behavioural Therapy (CBT) o   Group physical activity programmes

The IAPT (Improving Access to Psychological Therapies) programme has made these interventions more available in the last few years to people with milder cases of depression and anxiety, so that most no longer require referral to psychiatric services.

Cognitive Behavioural Therapy is a psychological intervention established by a psychiatrist called Aaron Beck. In summary, it is based on the understanding that negative thoughts and 'unhelpful' behaviours bring about a deterioration in mood (emotions), while actively making positive changes in thinking styles and behaviour result in corresponding improvements in mood. It has been found demonstrably effective in the treatment of many cases of depression and anxiety.

Antidepressants are only recommended in mild depression if symptoms have persisted for at least 2 years, do not respond to the above interventions, or the patient has previously suffered from moderate or severe depression. They can be initiated and monitored by the GP.

Moderate and severe depression:
These patients will usually be referred to a psychiatric service, and a combination of antidepressant medication and a high-intensity psychological intervention is recommended for their treatment.

Antidepressants

There are a number of classes of antidepressants, but those mostly used first-line are from the group called serotonin-specific reuptake inhibitors (SSRI's), examples of which include Sertraline, Fluoxetine, Citalopram and Escitalopram.

Antidepressants need to be taken every day to be effective, and will usually require about a fortnight to start exerting their effect on the mood. They need to be continued for at least 6 months after symptoms resolve, to reduce the risk of relapse. Depression is an illness that may prove recurrent in a number of people, and if there have been two or more severe depressive episodes in the recent past, antidepressants may need to be taken for 2 years at least.

They are not addictive medications, although some people may experience varying (usually non-severe) levels of discontinuation symptoms when they are stopped, especially if this is done abruptly without tapering off.

High-intensity psychological intervention

This could be cognitive behavioural therapy (CBT), interpersonal therapy (IPT), or other psychological therapies, dependent on what is available in the local psychiatric service.

Along with outpatient appointments with the psychiatrist, the above should be sufficient for most people being treated for depression by a psychiatric service, but other interventions that might be required (depending on need, illness severity and impairments in functioning) include:

Multidisciplinary team support

Support from a community psychiatric nurse (CPN), psychologist, occupational therapist and/or support worker might be offered if needed, in addition to clinic appointments.

Crisis or Home Treatment team support

This is an alternative to hospital admission, used when the patient is severely unwell and requires close monitoring, but their level of risk is low enough for them to be treated at home. The psychiatric home treatment team will visit daily, or a scheduled number of times a week, until the patient has made sufficient progress to be discharged from them and attend the outpatient clinic. They monitor the patient's risks, and often supervise them in taking their medication.

Inpatient treatment

This is required only in the most severe of cases of depression, for example if there is a significant risk of suicide, self-harm, severe self-neglect, or harm to others. Admission to the psychiatric ward will either be arranged on a voluntary basis (agreed to by the patient), or under a section of the Mental Health Act.

Electroconvulsive therapy (ECT)

This is used in severe cases of depression, where the condition has become life-threatening, or where other treatments have failed.

Resistant depression:

If depression proves resistant to antidepressant medication, a number of interventions can be used:

- Changing antidepressant (it may be helpful to try one in a different class).

- Adding CBT to the antidepressant.

- Adding another medication to the antidepressant, such as an antipsychotic, a second antidepressant, lithium (or other evidence-based recommended option).

Antipsychotic medication may be required particularly in cases of depression with psychotic features (delusions or hallucinations, as described above).

All patients being treated for depression will need ongoing monitoring and support from their GP, psychological or psychiatric service.

Psychoeducation will also be required (information given to the patient and their family/carers to help them better understand and manage the mental health problem and treatments).

N. I. Nwokolo

REFERENCES

1. Briers, S. (2012). *Brilliant Cognitive Behavioural Therapy: How to use CBT to improve your mind and your life*. UK: Pearson Education Limited.

2. Bullmore, E. (2018) *The Inflamed Mind: A Radical New Approach to Depression*. Short Books.

3. Cowen, P., Harrison, P., Burns, T. (2012) *Shorter Oxford Textbook of Psychiatry*. 6th ed. Oxford: Oxford University Press.

4. National Institute for Health and Care Excellence (2009) *The treatment and management of depression in adults* (update). NICE clinical guideline CG90.

5. Nwokolo, N. (2017) *Antipsychotics for Non-Psychotic Disorders: A Sample Mental Health Dissertation*. United Kingdom, CreateSpace Independent Publishing Platform.

6. Royal College of Psychiatrists (2014) *Depression: Key Facts*. RCPsych Public Education Editorial Board.

7. Semple, D., Smyth, R. (2013) *Oxford Handbook of Psychiatry*. Oxford: Oxford University Press.

8. World Health Organisation (1992) *The ICD-10 Classification of Mental and Behavioural Disorders: Clinical Descriptions and Diagnostic Guidelines*. Geneva: WHO.

N. I. Nwokolo

HELPFUL WEBSITES

Anxiety UK:
https://www.anxietyuk.org.uk

BACP Find a Therapist Directory:
https://www.bacp.co.uk/search/Therapists

Carers UK:
https://www.carersuk.org/Home

Depression Alliance:
https://www.depressionalliance.org

Mental health Foundation:
https://www.mentalhealth.org.uk

MIND:
https://www.mind.org.uk

National Institute for Health and Clinical Excellence:
https://www.NICE.org.uk

Rethink Mental Illness:
https://www.rethink.org

Royal College of Psychiatrists
https://www.rcpsych.ac.uk/

The Centre for Mental Health
https://www.centreformentalhealth.org.uk

ABOUT THE AUTHOR

The author is a UK psychiatrist, and works in the
National Health Service.